METABOLISM
AND YOU

Weight Loss
Guide
to Burning MORE Calories!

T. IRVOLINO

Copyright © 2019 by T. Irvolino
All rights reserved. No part of this book may be used or reproduced or transmitted in any form or by any means, electronic or mechanical including photocopying, recording, or by any information storage or retrieval system without express written permission from the publisher.

The information provided within this Book is for general informational purposes only. While we try to keep the information up-to-date and correct, there are no representations or warranties, express or implied, about the completeness, accuracy, reliability, suitability or availability with respect to the information, products, services, or related graphics contained in this Book for any purpose. Any use of this information is at your own risk.

The methods describe within this Book are the author's personal thoughts. They are not intended to be a definitive set of instructions for this project. You may discover there are other methods and materials to accomplish the same end result.

The author has made every effort to ensure the accuracy of the information within this book was correct at time of publication. The author and publisher do not assume and hereby disclaims any liability to any party for any loss, damage, or disruption caused by errors or omissions, whether such errors or omissions result from accident, negligence, or any other cause.

Sun Media Group, LLC
First Book Publication Date: 1/2019
Cover Illustration: T. Irvolino
To contact Author, please email publisher: sunmediagroupllc@gmail.com

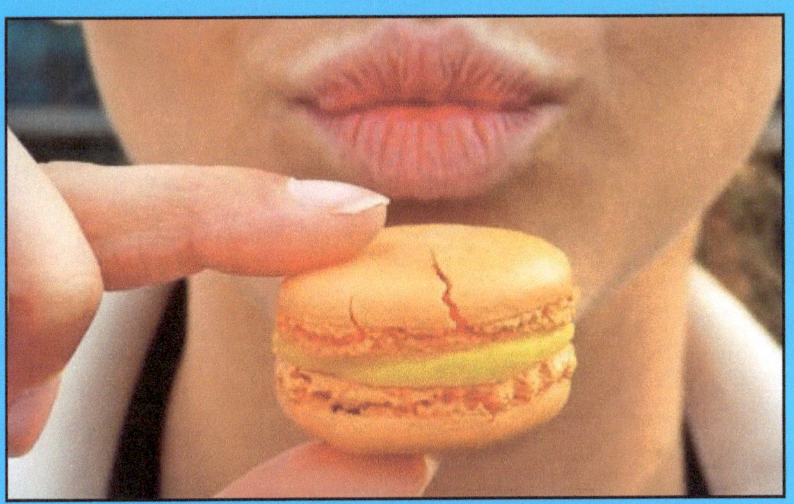

As we all know too well, your body needs calories to keep you going every day. The food you eat turns into fuel to get you through your day.

Your metabolism is the key to converting food into energy. It is the process by which your body converts what you eat and drink into energy. During this complex biochemical process, calories in food and beverages are combined with oxygen to release the energy your body needs to function.

Diet and exercise is an everlasting process to help you maintain your desired weight. The key to weight-loss is boosting your metabolism to help aid in the process.

01

What is Metabolism?

Metabolism is the process by which your body converts what you eat and drink into energy. During this complex biochemical process, calories in food and beverages are combined with oxygen to release the energy your body needs to function. Whether you're sleeping, running, sitting, standing, or riding in a car your body is constantly burning calories in order to keep you going.

As we age, our metabolism slows down. Our bodies don't contain as much muscle mass at the age of 60 than we do at the age of 20. Muscle mass is a key factor to help burn those added calories.

Everyone is different. Some people have higher metabolisms and are able to burn off the calories they eat and never gain an ounce. Others have slower metabolisms and everything they eat seems pack on the pounds. No two people are alike in the calories they burn and the rate their metabolism uses those calories for fuel.

As we go forward, keep in mind of your age and activity level now, verses little ideas that will help you boost your metabolism for added weight loss and overall greater health.

Evidence suggests that there are a number of ways to help augment your metabolism in order to more efficiently consume the right foods at the right time of the day. Whether you're walking, reading or even sleeping, boosting your metabolic rate is possible and I'll show you how.

02

Dieting... Do's and Don't

To lose a pound of fat, you have to burn 3,500 calories more than you consume, so you can see how hard it is to exercise your way through a poor diet. Instead, you have to watch what you eat.

Like everyone I know, the word diet means no food, no fun! Life as you know it would drastically change and so would your social life.

Example:
I can't go out, I'm on a diet...

....and the age old, you tell your family and friends, you are dieting and they see you eating a cookie...

Why are you eating that, I thought you were on a diet!

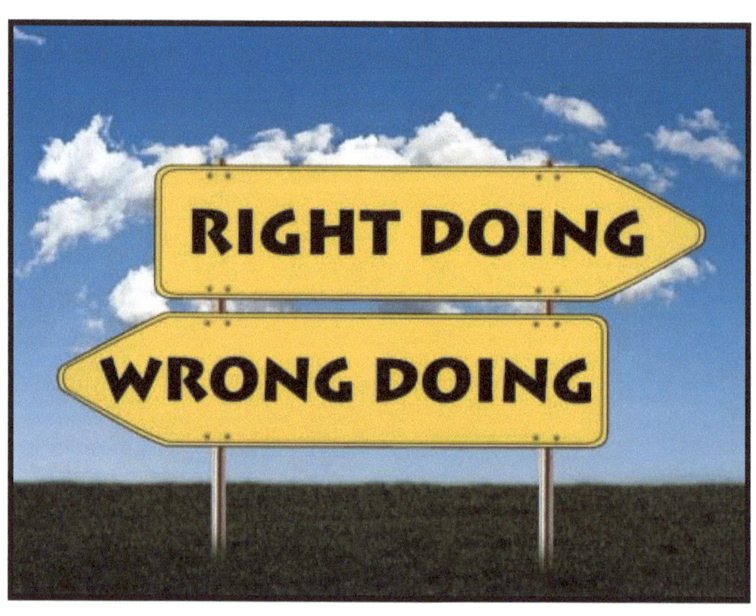

RIGHT DOING
WRONG DOING

Automatically, your body goes into defense mode mentally and physically. You just told yourself that the cookie is going to make you gain weight, even though it makes you feel better. Our bodies are very efficient at storing food as fat as a defense against starvation. When you cut your calories, and if you do it drastically enough, your body panics.

If you shock your body with lack of calories, it kicks your metabolism into slow mode. Instead of burning those calories for fuel, it burns muscle. The less muscle mass you have, the less calories you burn. This means that if you consume more calories, your body won't need to use them for energy and will store them.

Once off your diet, the weight will return as fat and stored. Every time you crash diet you are slowing your metabolism over and over. Here, you will learn to increase your metabolism in order to burn the most calories possible, even when sleeping.

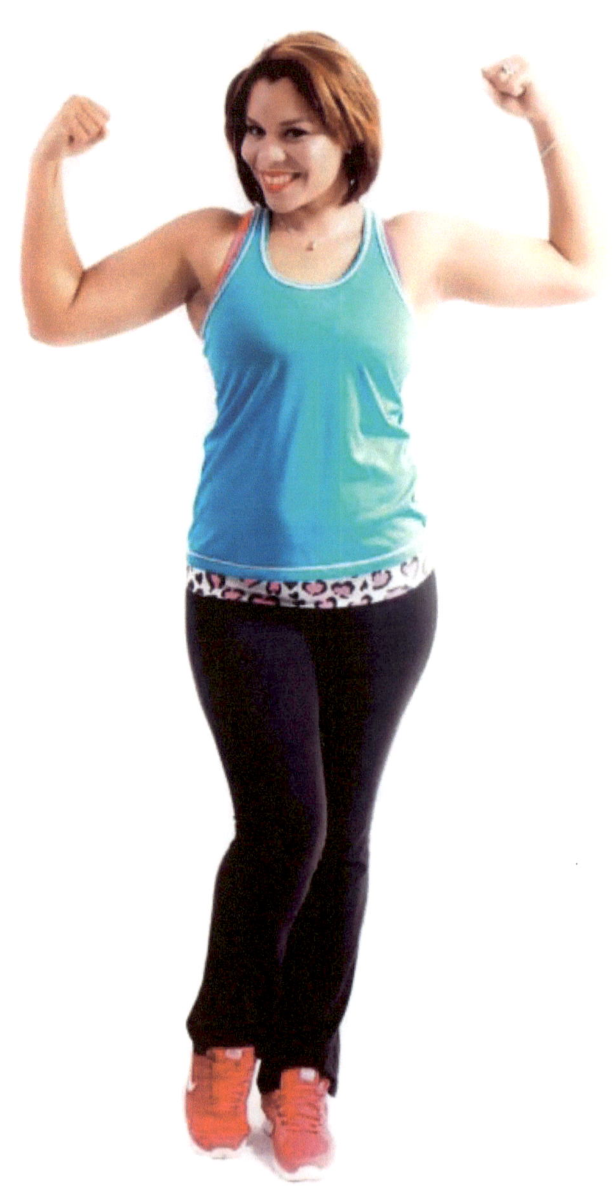

03

Boosting your Metabolism

If you want to boost your metabolism, the best thing you can do is begin exercising.

Strength Training. Some exercise is good for building muscle and some is good for just plain sweating. Strength training is a type of exercise that requires you to contract your muscles against resistance. You create that resistance and put your muscles to work by using hand-held weights, weight machines, resistance bands, resistance balls and even your own body resistance.

While aerobic exercises like jogging, playing tennis or riding a bike will help you tone your body and maintain your weight, they don't do a whole lot to increase your muscle mass which is what you need to do in order to boost your metabolism.

How Strength Training Benefits Your Health

- Strength training makes you stronger and fitter

- Strength training protects bone health and muscle mass

- Strength training helps keep the weight off for good

- Strength training helps you develop better body mechanics

- Strength training can help with chronic disease management

As you increase your muscle mass, your stored fat decreases and your metabolism increases. It burns more calories of what you eat.

Your body will require more calories to maintain itself. By increasing your muscle mass through weight and strength training, and consuming a lower caloric intake daily, **YOU WILL LOSE WEIGHT**. Just don't lower your calories so drastically that it sends your body into survival mode again.

Boosting your metabolism through exercise is just one way to burn those calories.

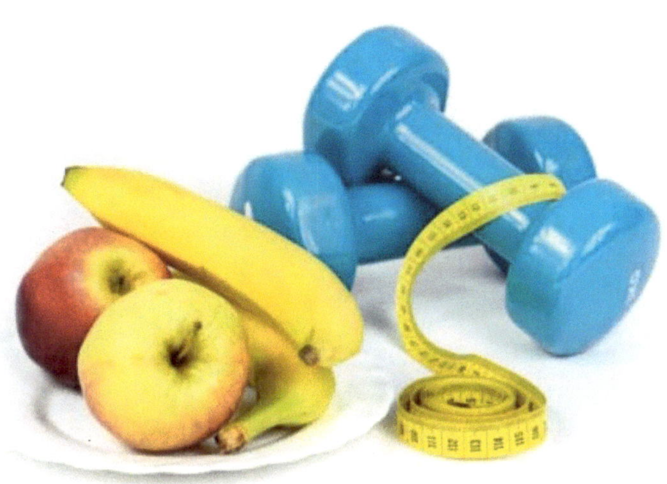

3 Meals per Day vs. 6 Smaller Meals per Day

Morning

Slows Metabolism
Poor Food Choices for the rest of the Day

Noon

Over Tired and Sluggish
Loss of Concentration

Night

Craving More Carbs
No Energy - Late Night Hunger

Raises Metabolism
Healthy Choices for the rest of the Day

Full of Energy
Never Hungry

Rapid Weight Loss

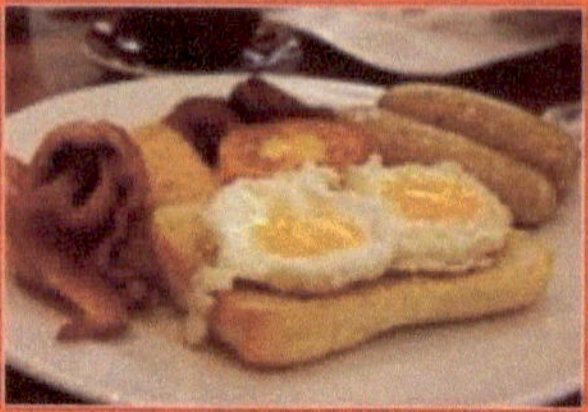

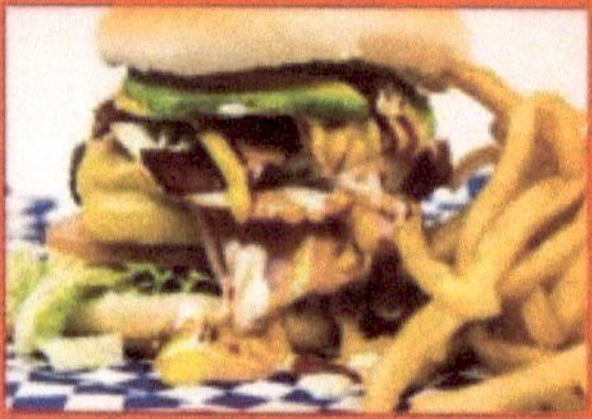

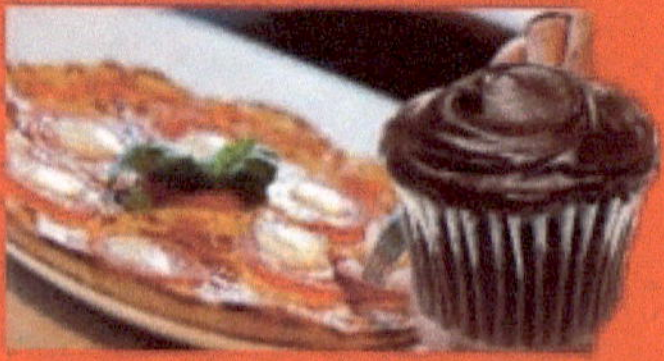

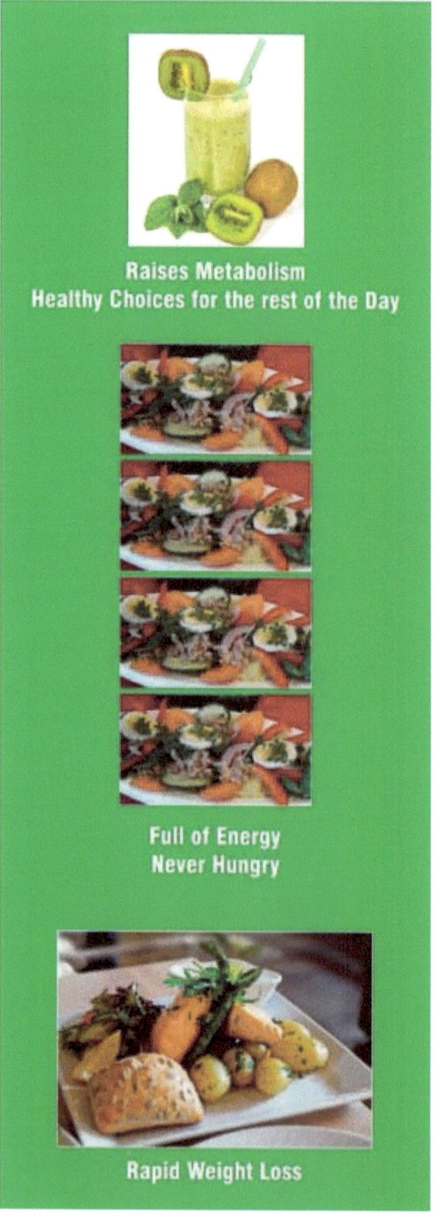

04

Daily Food Intake

YOU MUST EAT!!! You have to eat in order to keep your metabolism running in an optimal manner.

How many of us skip meals to save on calories? Everyone! That is not the way to go. As you skip a meal, your body is saying, OMG! we didn't get any food, we need to save what's there to survive!

Remember, not eating sends signals to your body that you are starving and kicks your metabolism into overdrive. It slows down the burning of caloric intake and stores it for future use, as fat. Especially in the morning. After sleeping all night, you wake up and your body is looking for nourishment to get your metabolism working. It can go both ways. Either you eat or we will store fat.

Having a good healthy breakfast will jump start

your body into burning calories, rather than storage.

Eat small meals and eat them often during the day.

Research has shown that breaking down the traditional three meals a day into six smaller meals, spaced evenly throughout the day will result in a boost to your metabolism.

Of course you need to be aware of what you are eating.

Mix up your morning meal and try one - or a few of these 5 healthy breakfast foods that help you lose weight.

- Raspberries
- Oatmeal
- Yogurt
- Peanut Butter
- Eggs

Break your meals into six smaller and healthier meals. Lowering your caloric intake in a healthy manner will not only make you feel more energized, it will give your metabolism a great jump start to your day.

Eat more complex carbohydrates. They take a longer time to be absorbed into your body and this enables your blood sugar to remain level.

Nutrient-dense complex carbs that are part of a healthy, balanced diet include:

- Whole wheat breads, pastas, and flour.
- Brown and wild rices
- Barley
- Quinoa
- Potatoes
- Corn
- Legumes, such as black beans, chickpeas, lentils, etc.

Avoid simple sugars, rice and refined flour which are all absorbed quickly by your body and are turned into fat.

QUESTION: YES OR NO?
Can coffee make you put on weight? Be mindful...

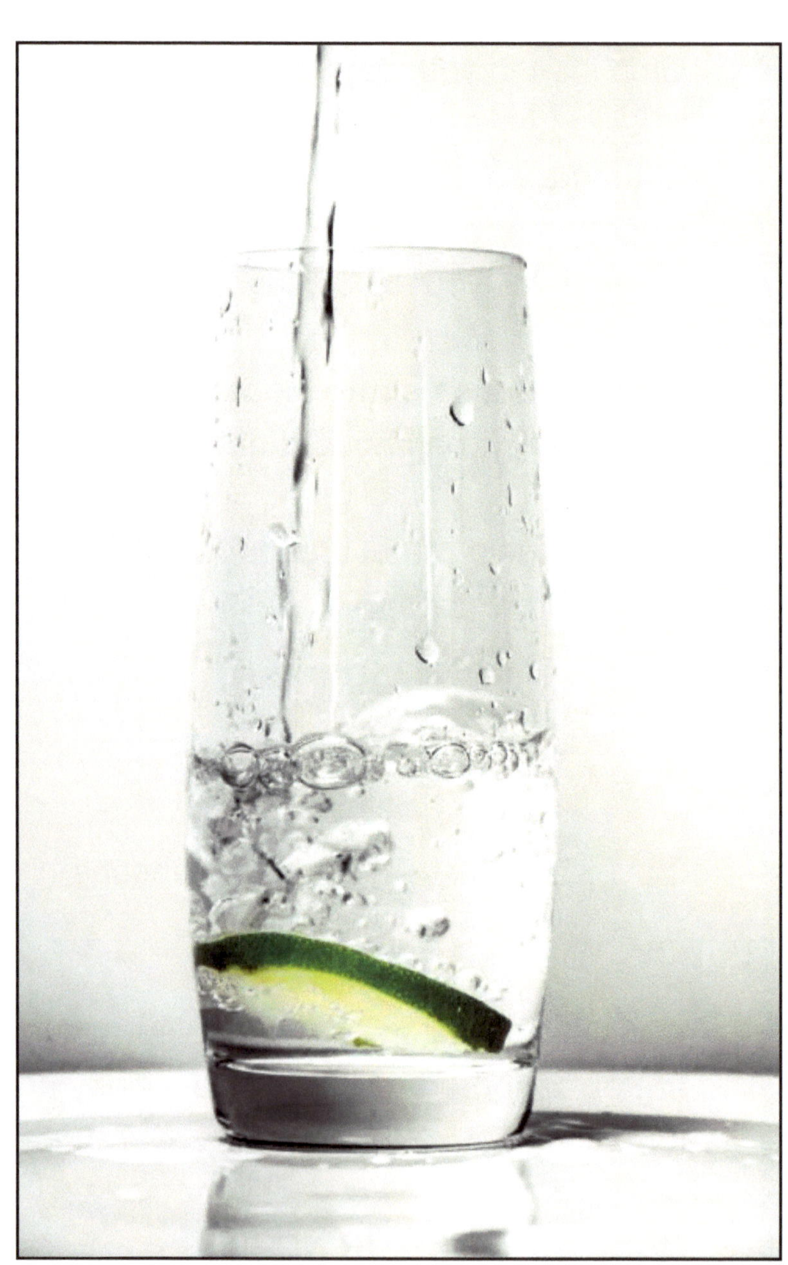

Starting your day with a caffeine buzz isn't likely to cause weight gain -- coffee served black is low in calories. But overdoing it can make you pack on the pounds, especially if your beverage contains added sugar and milk. If you need that cup of coffee in the morning, have it. This isn't a diet, it's a life change.

Green tea is a good alternative. It's high in antioxidants. Caffeine is known to block absorption of vitamin C, create a bit of unhealthy acid in your system and stimulate sugar cravings. If there's one thing you don't need when you're trying to lose weight, its sugar cravings.

Try to drink at least 8 glasses of water daily. Water cleans out all the toxins when you're losing weight. If you are becoming dehydrated your metabolism will slow down. Try drinking ice cold water. Your body should remain warm and it will boost your metabolism a bit each time it has to warm up.

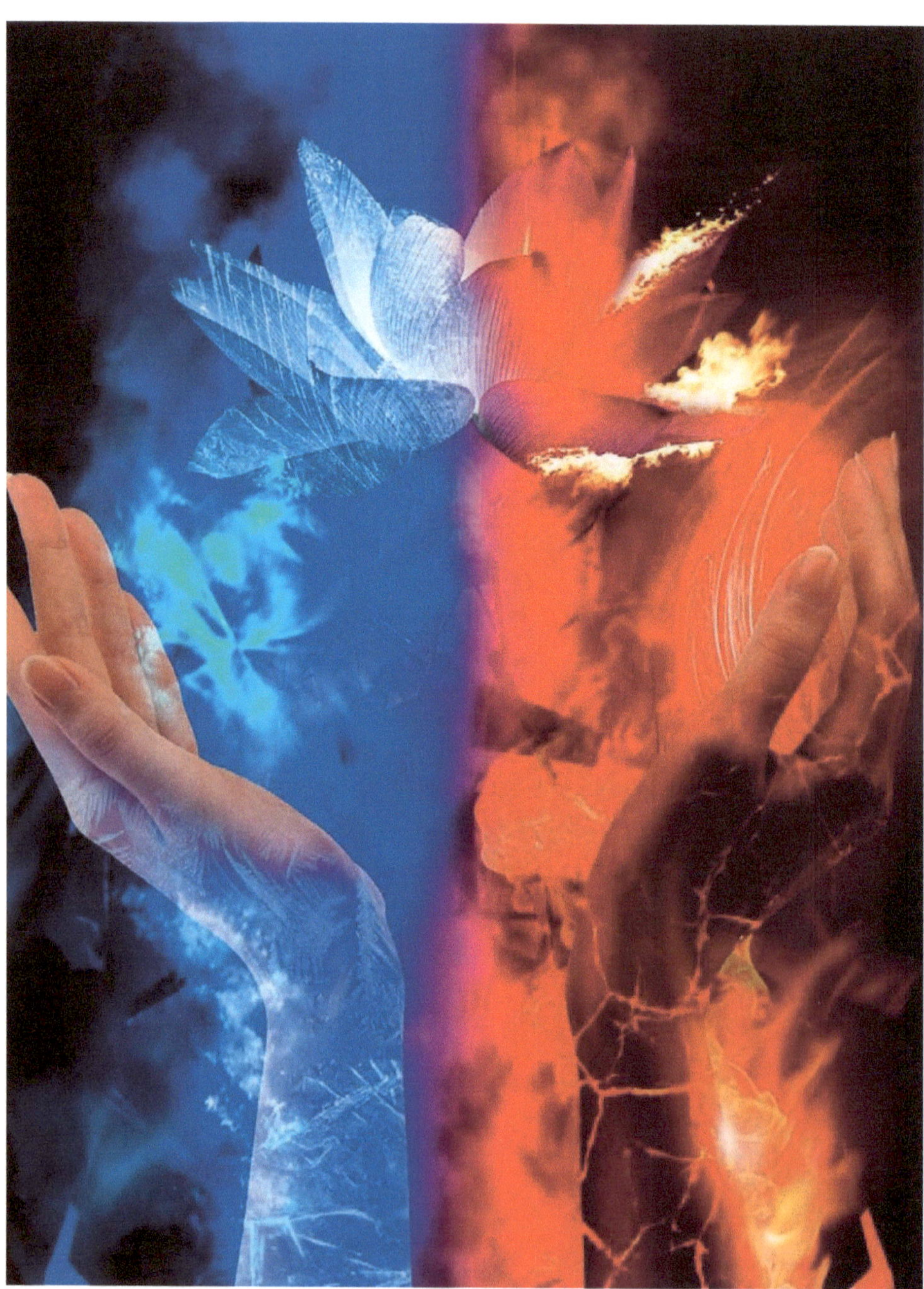

05

Other Methods to Boost your Metabolism

Lowering or raising your body temperature has shown to boost your metabolism by about 20%. Soak in a nice warm tub or spend some time in a sauna. Take a short brisk walk in the winter. Heating yourself up and cooling off may just help.

Another way to give yourself a boost, add some spice to your life. Studies have shown that eating spicy foods with cayenne pepper, jalapeño or chili peppers will give a boost to your metabolism as well.

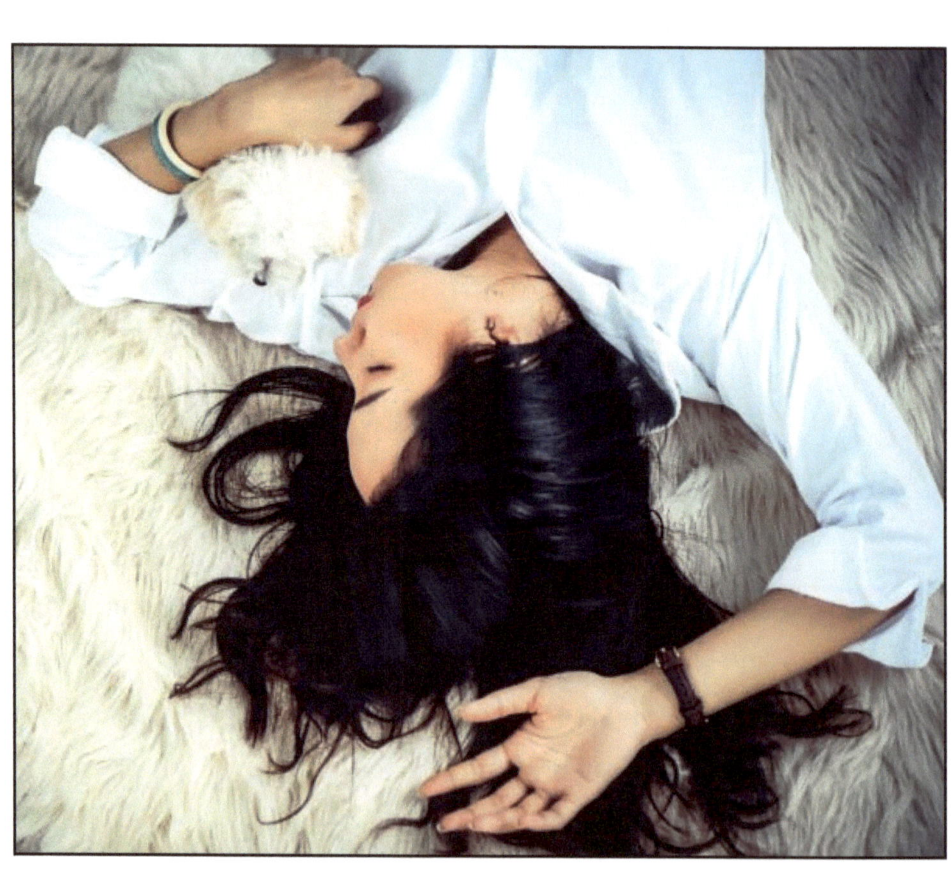

06

Sleep

Your metabolism naturally slows down during the night, especially because you're most likely sleeping and not actively exercising, doing chores or eating food. Night is a time that your body rests so it has a chance to repair tissue, improve cognitive function and restore energy levels.

Why Sleep Is Important for Weight Loss.

People who are sleep deprived tend to weigh more and have more trouble losing weight than those who get adequate rest, even when they follow the same diet. When you don't get enough sleep, your body over produces the hunger causing hormones leptin and ghrelin.

While you're resting, you're avoiding stress. Stress is known to increase your chances of gaining weight. Stress releases a steroid called cortisol which depresses your metabolism, thereby encouraging your body to conserve calories as fat. Avoid stress at all costs.

07

Conclusion

There are so many thing to consider while trying to lose weight. First and foremost, before starting any diet or weight-loss program, you need to speak with your doctor for advice. Remember, everyone is different and each person will lose weight at a different speed.

This e-book is to inform you of how important your metabolism is for wight loss. Increasing your metabolism means not starving yourself, build muscle mass, eat small meals throughout the day and avoiding stress.

Daily Checklist

Date:

✓	Today's To Do List

Today's Meal Plan
Breakfast - Lunch - Dinner

Food Journal

	Food / Beverage	Calories
Breakfast		
Lunch		
Dinner		
Snacks		

Total Calories	

Exercise Routine		# Minutes

Water Intake Checklist	

Daily Checklist

Date:

✓	Today's To Do List

Today's Meal Plan
Breakfast – Lunch – Dinner

Food Journal

	Food / Beverage	Calories
Breakfast		
Lunch		
Dinner		
Snacks		

Total Calories	

Exercise Routine		# Minutes

Water Intake Checklist	

Daily Checklist

Date:

✓	Today's To Do List

Today's Meal Plan
Breakfast - Lunch - Dinner

Food Journal

	Food / Beverage	Calories
Breakfast		
Lunch		
Dinner		
Snacks		

Total Calories	

Exercise Routine		# Minutes

Water Intake Checklist	

www.ingramcontent.com/pod-product-compliance
Lightning Source LLC
Chambersburg PA
CBHW040252240726
48664CB00001B/368